LOW SODIUM COOKBOOK FOR SENIORS

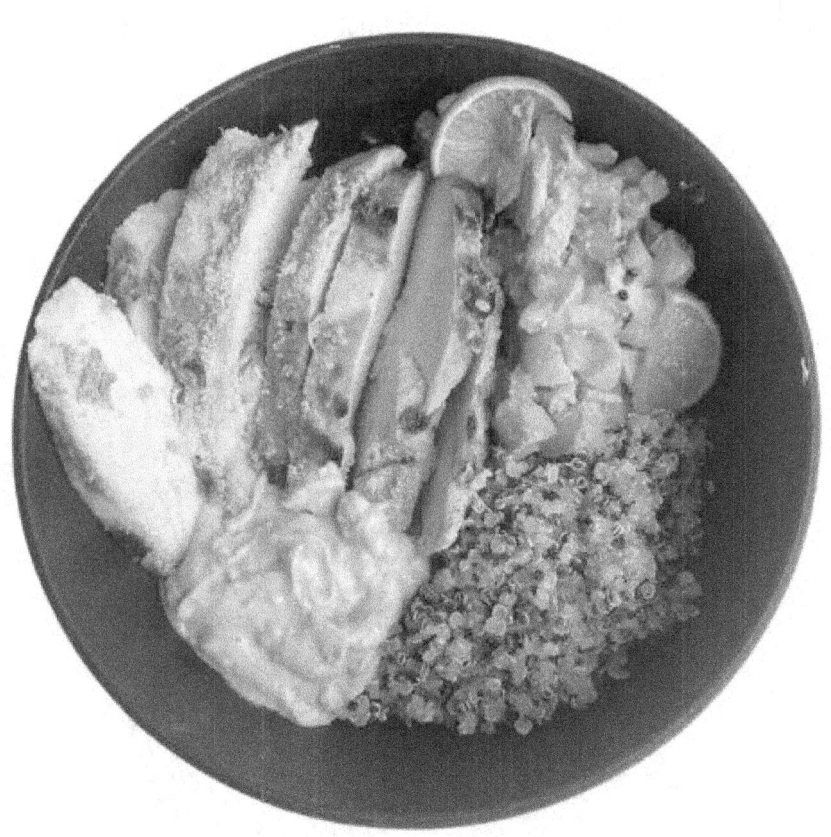

LORENE PEACHEY

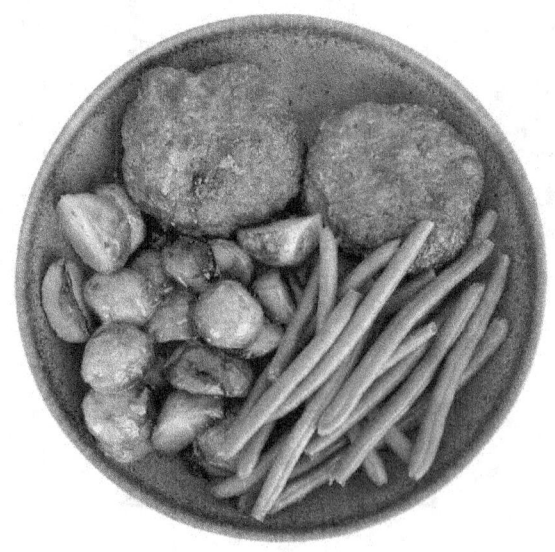

TABLE OF CONTENTS

INTRODUCTION

In the quiet town of Harmony Ville, I met Mr. Emerson Wilkerson, a charming octogenarian with a love for life that surpassed his years. Known for his infectious laughter and a twinkle in his eye that hinted at a lifetime of stories, Mr. Wilkerson had faced a health challenge that threatened to dim his vibrant spirit.

My journey with Mr. Wilkerson began when he walked into my nutrition clinic one gloomy Tuesday afternoon. He had a stack of cookbooks under his arm, a testament to his quest for a solution. "Lorene Peachey, Nutritionist Extraordinaire" was emblazoned across the covers of those books – my previous attempts to guide him toward a healthier lifestyle.

As a seasoned nutritionist, I had crafted meal plans and recipes, carefully selecting ingredients to promote well-being. However, despite our shared enthusiasm, Mr. Wilkerson's health remained stagnant. It was clear that something needed to change.

One day, he walked into my office, a gleam of hope in his eyes. "Lorene," he said, "I've tried it all, and nothing seems to work. I feel like I'm running out of options. "My heart sank, but the determined glint in his eye challenged me to find a solution. I took a deep breath and shared with him a secret weapon I had been saving for just the right moment – my very own cookbook, "Low Sodium Cookbook for Seniors."

The transformation that unfolded in Mr. Wilkerson's life was nothing short of remarkable. "Lorene, these recipes have breathed life back into my kitchen," he exclaimed. "I'm feeling better, more energetic. I can taste the Flavors without worrying about my sodium intake!"

This cookbook, born out of a passion for promoting healthy living among seniors, became a beacon of culinary hope for Mr. Wilkerson. But what made " Low Sodium Cookbook for Seniors " stand out from the sea of cookbooks he had tried before?

As we delved into the recipes, Mr. Wilkerson and I discovered a symphony of Flavors that surpassed his expectations. From savory Baked Zucchini Boats with Turkey to the delightful Creamy Avocado Banana Smoothie, every recipe was crafted with care and creativity. "These aren't just meals; they're experiences," he chuckled between bites of a heartwarming Sweet Potato and Black Bean Chili.

The benefits of a low-sodium diet for seniors are vast, and they became glaringly evident in Mr. Wilkerson's life. Reduced sodium intake can lead to lower blood pressure, alleviating the strain on the heart. The risk of heart disease, a concern for many seniors, diminishes when sodium is kept in check. I watched as Mr. Wilkerson's vitality returned, a testament to the power of mindful eating.

"Do you remember the last time you felt truly alive?" I asked him during one of our consultations. His eyes sparkled as he recalled a vivid memory of a summer picnic from decades past. "That's the feeling we're aiming for," I grinned, knowing that " Low Sodium Cookbook for Seniors " was steering him toward that very destination.

High sodium levels have consequences, and Mr. Wilkerson's journey shed light on this reality. High blood pressure, kidney damage, and an increased risk of stroke are just a few of the unwelcome outcomes that a diet rich in sodium can bring. As we flipped through the pages of my cookbook, the contrast between his past struggles and the newfound vibrancy of his life became glaringly apparent.

" Low Sodium Cookbook for Seniors " extends beyond just a collection of recipes; it's a guide to a rejuvenated life. The advantage lies not only in the delicious and wholesome meals but also in the holistic approach to well-being.

The friendly tone of the cookbook resonates with seniors, making the journey towards a low-sodium lifestyle both enjoyable and attainable.

As Mr. Wilkerson embraced this culinary adventure, he rediscovered the joy of cooking and the pleasures of sharing a meal with loved ones. "I never thought healthy eating could taste this good!" he chuckled, savouring the Flavors of a delectable Balsamic Glazed Chicken with Roasted Vegetables.

The benefits of a low-sodium diet for seniors extend beyond the physical. The emotional connection to food is profound, and " Low Sodium Cookbook for Seniors " taps into this sentiment. It became not just a cookbook but a companion on Mr. Wilkerson's journey to better health. The simple act of flipping through its pages evoked memories, stirred creativity, and brought a renewed sense of purpose to his culinary endeavours.

As you embark on this gastronomic journey with " Low Sodium Cookbook for Seniors," consider the questions that lie within your own story. What memories do you want to create around your dining table? How do you envision your health in the coming years? Can you imagine the delight of savouring a delicious, low-sodium dessert without compromising your well-being?

This cookbook isn't just a guide; it's an invitation to a life of flavour, health, and joy. It's a reminder that every meal is an opportunity to nourish not only your body but also your soul. So, my dear reader, are you ready to Savor the harmony of a low-sodium life?

" Low Sodium Cookbook for Seniors " isn't just a cookbook – it's a culinary journey toward a healthier, happier you. As you turn the pages, let the aroma of fresh ingredients and the promise of delightful Flavors inspire you. Embrace the transformation, Savor the moments, and let the symphony of low-sodium goodness lead you to a life of vitality and fulfillment.

Welcome to "" Low Sodium Cookbook for Seniors," where every meal is a celebration of health, happiness, and the sheer joy of living.

Contact the Author

Thank you for reading my book! I would love to hear from you, whether you have feedback, questions, or just want to share your thoughts. Your feedback means a lot to me and helps me improve as a writer.

Please don't hesitate to reach out to me through

lorenepeachey@gmail.com

I look forward to connecting with my readers and appreciate your support in this literary journey. Your thoughts and comments are valuable to me.

CHAPTER 1

UNDERSTANDING SODIUM

Sodium is a vital mineral that plays a crucial role in maintaining the balance of fluids in and around cells, as well as in nerve function and muscle contraction. It is an essential electrolyte, working in tandem with potassium to regulate water balance and support various physiological processes in the body.

The Role of Sodium in the Body

Fluid Balance: Sodium helps regulate the balance of fluids both inside and outside cells. This balance is critical for proper cell function, blood pressure regulation, and overall hydration.

Nerve Function: Sodium is essential for transmitting nerve impulses. Nerve cells, or neurons, rely on the movement of sodium ions to generate electrical signals, facilitating communication between different parts of the nervous system.

Muscle Contraction: Sodium is involved in the process of muscle contraction. It works alongside potassium to maintain the electrical charge necessary for muscle cells to contract and relax.

pH Regulation: Sodium plays a role in maintaining the body's acid-base balance, helping to regulate the pH of bodily fluids.

Recommended Daily Sodium Intake for Seniors

While sodium is essential for health, excessive intake can contribute to health issues, especially for seniors. The recommended daily sodium intake for seniors is generally around 1,200 to 1,500 milligrams. However, individual needs may vary based on factors like health status and activity level.

Seniors are often advised to limit sodium intake to help manage conditions such as high blood pressure, kidney disease, and cardiovascular issues. It's essential for seniors to focus on a balanced diet with fresh fruits, vegetables, lean proteins, and whole grains while minimizing processed and packaged foods high in sodium.

Hidden Sources of Sodium in Foods

Many foods contain hidden sources of sodium, and being aware of these is crucial for maintaining a healthy diet:

Processed Foods: Packaged and processed foods, including canned soups, frozen meals, and snacks, often contain high levels of sodium for flavor enhancement and preservation.

Condiments and Sauces: Common condiments like soy sauce, ketchup, and salad dressings can be surprisingly high in sodium. Opt for low-sodium alternatives or use herbs and spices for flavoring.

Cured and Smoked Meats: Bacon, ham, and smoked meats are examples of foods that can be rich in sodium due to the curing and smoking processes.

Cheese: Certain types of cheese, especially processed varieties, can contribute significant amounts of sodium to your diet.

Bakery Products: Some baked goods, such as bread and pastries, may contain hidden sodium, so it's advisable to check labels and choose low-sodium options.

CHAPTER 2

GETTING STARTED

Stocking a Low Sodium Pantry

Creating a low-sodium pantry is a key step in managing sodium intake and promoting overall health. Here are some tips for stocking a pantry with low-sodium options:

Whole Grains: Choose whole grains such as brown rice, quinoa, and whole wheat pasta. These provide essential nutrients without the added sodium found in some processed grains.

Canned Goods: Opt for low-sodium or no-salt-added canned goods, including beans, vegetables, and tomatoes. Rinse canned beans and vegetables to further reduce sodium content.

Herbs and Spices: Build a collection of herbs and spices to add flavor to your dishes without relying on salt. Popular choices include basil, oregano, garlic powder, onion powder, and cumin.

Low-Sodium Broths: Keep low-sodium chicken, vegetable, or beef broths on hand for soups, stews, and cooking grains. Be sure to check labels to find options with reduced sodium content.

Oils and Vinegars: Use olive oil, canola oil, and various vinegars to enhance the taste of your meals without relying on salt. Experiment with balsamic vinegar, red wine vinegar, and apple cider vinegar for different flavors.

Nuts and Seeds: Include unsalted nuts and seeds in your pantry, such as almonds, walnuts, chia seeds, and flaxseeds. They add crunch and nutrition without excess sodium.

Dried Herbs and Garlic: Keep a stock of dried herbs, such as thyme, rosemary, and sage, as well as garlic and onion powder. These can be used in cooking or as toppings for various dishes.

Low-Sodium Sauces: Look for low-sodium soy sauce, tamari, and other sauces to add depth to your recipes. Be cautious with condiments, as they can be a hidden source of sodium.

Reading Food Labels Effectively

Understanding food labels is crucial for identifying and managing sodium intake. Here are some tips for reading food labels effectively:

Serving Size Awareness: Pay attention to the serving size listed on the label, as this can significantly impact the amount of sodium you consume.

Sodium Content: Check the sodium content per serving. Products labeled as "low sodium" typically contain 140 milligrams or less per serving.

% Daily Value (%DV): Use the %DV to gauge how much a serving of the product contributes to your daily sodium intake. Aim for foods with lower percentages.

Ingredients List: Examine the ingredients list for terms related to sodium, such as sodium chloride, monosodium glutamate (MSG), and sodium bicarbonate. Be cautious of hidden sources of sodium.

Compare Products: When choosing between similar products, compare their sodium content to make the best low-sodium choices.

Cooking Techniques for Flavor without Salt

Cooking without salt doesn't mean sacrificing flavor. Try these techniques to enhance taste without relying on sodium:

Herbs and Spices: Experiment with a variety of herbs and spices to add depth and complexity to your dishes. Fresh herbs like basil, cilantro, and thyme can elevate the flavors.

Citrus Juices: Use citrus juices such as lemon or lime to brighten up the taste of salads, vegetables, and proteins.

Vinegars: Different types of vinegars, such as balsamic or apple cider vinegar, can provide acidity and flavor to your meals.

Garlic and Onions: Incorporate fresh garlic and onions into your recipes to impart robust and savory notes to your dishes.

Grilling and Roasting: Grilling and roasting intensify the natural flavors of ingredients, adding depth without the need for excessive salt.

Broths and Stocks: Opt for low-sodium or homemade broths and stocks to enhance the taste of soups, stews, and sauces.

Marinating: Marinate proteins in flavorful mixtures with herbs, spices, and acids like vinegar or citrus juices to infuse taste without relying on salt.

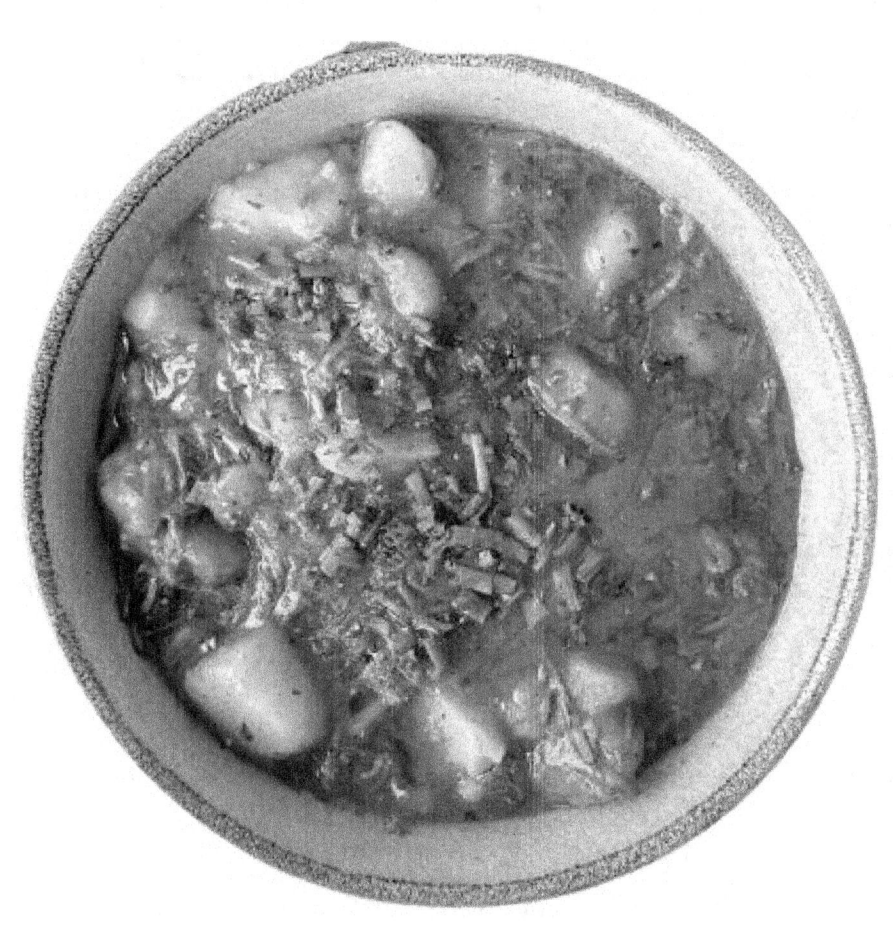

CHAPTER 3

BREAKFAST DELIGHTS

Vegetable Omelets

Cooking Time: 10 minutes | Serving: 1

Ingredients:

- ❖ 2 eggs
- ❖ Assorted vegetables (bell peppers, tomatoes, spinach)
- ❖ Olive oil
- ❖ Herbs and spices (chives, thyme)
- ❖ Salt-free seasoning

Instructions:

1. Whisk eggs in a bowl.
2. Sauté chopped vegetables in olive oil.
3. Pour eggs over veggies, add herbs, and cook until set.
4. Season with salt-free seasoning.

Nutritional Information:

220 calories, 12g carbs, 14g protein, 14g fat, 3g fiber.

Start your day with a nutrient-packed omelette, rich in protein and veggies, supporting energy and vitality.

Greek Yogurt Parfait

Prep Time: 5 minutes | Serving: 1

Ingredients:

- ❖ 1 cup plain Greek yogurt
- ❖ Fresh berries (blueberries, strawberries)
- ❖ Almonds (chopped)
- ❖ Honey (optional)

Instructions:

1. Layer yogurt with berries in a glass.
2. Top with chopped almonds and drizzle with honey.

Nutritional Information:

250 calories, 20g carbs, 15g protein, 12g fat, 5g fiber.

Indulge in a delightful parfait, offering a protein boost from Greek yogurt and antioxidants from

Avocado Toast with Tomato

Prep Time: 7 minutes | Serving: 1

Ingredients:

- ❖ 1 slice whole-grain bread
- ❖ 1/2 ripe avocado
- ❖ Sliced tomatoes.
- ❖ Red pepper flakes
- ❖ Fresh lemon juice

Instructions:

1. Toast the whole-grain bread.
2. Mash the avocado and spread it on the toast.
3. Top with sliced tomatoes, a dash of red pepper flakes, and a squeeze of fresh lemon juice.

Nutritional Information:

220 calories, 20g carbs, 5g protein, 15g fat, 7g fiber.

Enjoy a heart-healthy breakfast with the creamy goodness of avocado, paired with the freshness of tomatoes.

Quinoa Breakfast Bowl

Cooking Time: 15 minutes | Serving: 1

Ingredients:

- ❖ 1/2 cup cooked quinoa
- ❖ Greek yogurt
- ❖ Fresh fruits (banana slices, berries)
- ❖ Nuts (walnuts or almonds)
- ❖ Drizzle of maple syrup

Instructions:

1. Mix cooked quinoa with Greek yogurt.
2. Top with fresh fruits and nuts.
3. Drizzle with a touch of maple syrup.

Nutritional Information:

280 calories, 40g carbs, 12g protein, 8g fat, 6g fiber.

Elevate your morning with a protein-packed quinoa bowl, offering a delightful blend of textures and flavors.

Apple Cinnamon Chia Pudding

Prep Time: 5 minutes (plus chilling time) | Serving: 1

Ingredients:

- ❖ 2 tbsp chia seeds
- ❖ 1/2 cup unsweetened almond milk
- ❖ 1/2 apple (diced)
- ❖ Cinnamon
- ❖ Drizzle of honey

Instructions:

1. Mix chia seeds with almond milk and let it sit in the fridge for at least 2 hours or overnight.
2. Layer diced apples on top, sprinkle with cinnamon, and drizzle with honey.

Nutritional Information:

220 calories, 25g carbs, 6g protein, 12g fat, 8g fiber.

Savor a nutritious chia pudding loaded with omega-3s, fiber, and the natural sweetness of apples.

Banana Nut Smoothie Bowl

Prep Time: 8 minutes | Serving: 1

Ingredients:

- ❖ 1 ripe banana
- ❖ 1/2 cup low-fat yogurt
- ❖ Handful of mixed nuts (walnuts, almonds)
- ❖ Chia seeds
- ❖ Drizzle of honey

Instructions:

1. Blend banana and yogurt until smooth.
2. Pour into a bowl and top with mixed nuts, chia seeds, and a drizzle of honey.

Nutritional Information:

260 calories, 30g carbs, 10g protein, 12g fat, 5g fiber.

Delight in a creamy and satisfying smoothie bowl, brimming with potassium from bananas and the crunch of nutrient-packed nuts.

Spinach and Feta Breakfast Wrap

Cooking Time: 10 minutes | Serving: 1

Ingredients:

- ❖ 1 whole-grain wrap
- ❖ Handful of fresh spinach
- ❖ 2 eggs (scrambled)
- ❖ Feta cheese (crumbled)
- ❖ Salsa (optional)

Instructions:

1. Sauté fresh spinach until wilted.
2. Scramble eggs and fold in feta cheese.
3. Fill the wrap with the egg mixture and top with salsa if desired.

Nutritional Information:

300 calories, 25g carbs, 18g protein, 14g fat, 6g fiber.

Kickstart your day with a savory breakfast wrap, featuring the goodness of leafy greens and protein-packed eggs.

Blueberry Almond Overnight Oats

Prep Time: 5 minutes (plus chilling time) | Serving: 1

Ingredients:

- ❖ 1/2 cup rolled oats.
- ❖ 1/2 cup unsweetened almond milk
- ❖ Fresh blueberries
- ❖ Almond slices
- ❖ Drizzle of agave syrup

Instructions:

1. Mix oats and almond milk, let it refrigerate overnight.
2. Top with fresh blueberries, almond slices, and a drizzle of agave syrup.

Nutritional Information:

240 calories, 35g carbs, 7g protein, 8g fat, 5g fiber.

Indulge in the convenience of overnight oats, offering a delightful blend of fiber, antioxidants, and crunch.

Sweet Potato and Turkey Hash

Cooking Time: 15 minutes | Serving: 1

Ingredients:

- ❖ 1 small, sweet potato (diced)
- ❖ Lean ground turkey
- ❖ Onion (chopped)
- ❖ Bell peppers (sliced)
- ❖ Smoked paprika and black pepper.

Instructions:

1. Sauté sweet potatoes until slightly crispy.
2. Add ground turkey, onion, and bell peppers.
3. Season with smoked paprika and black pepper.

Nutritional Information:

280 calories, 30g carbs, 20g protein, 10g fat, 6g fiber.

Fuel your morning with a protein-packed sweet potato and turkey hash, providing a savory and satisfying start.

Coconut Mango Chia Pudding Bowl

Prep Time: 5 minutes (plus chilling time) | Serving: 1

Ingredients:

- ❖ 2 tbsp chia seeds
- ❖ 1/2 cup coconut milk
- ❖ Fresh mango chunks
- ❖ Unsweetened shredded coconut
- ❖ Mint leaves for garnish

Instructions:

1. Mix chia seeds with coconut milk and refrigerate until set.
2. Top with fresh mango chunks, shredded coconut, and mint leaves.

Nutritional Information:

250 calories, 30g carbs, 6g protein, 12g fat, 8g fiber.

Indulge in a tropical chia pudding bowl, a refreshing and nutritious way to start your day.

These breakfast recipes offer a variety of flavors, textures, and nutrients, ensuring a satisfying and health-conscious start to your day. Each recipe is carefully crafted to be low in sodium, catering to the specific dietary needs of seniors. Remember, a nutritious breakfast sets the stage for a day filled with energy, positivity, and well-being.

CHAPTER 4

HEART-HEALTHY SOUPS

Lentil and Vegetable Soup

Cooking Time: 45 minutes | Serving: 4

Ingredients:

- ❖ 1 cup dried lentils
- ❖ Mixed vegetables (carrots, celery, onion)
- ❖ Low-sodium vegetable broth
- ❖ Garlic, thyme, bay leaves
- ❖ Spinach leaves

Instructions:

1. Sauté garlic, add vegetables, and cook until softened.
2. Stir in lentils, broth, and herbs. Simmer until lentils are tender.
3. Add spinach before serving.

Nutritional Information:

180 calories, 30g carbs, 12g protein, 1g fat, 8g fiber.

Enjoy a hearty lentil soup rich in fiber and plant-based protein, supporting heart health and providing essential nutrients.

Tomato Basil Quinoa Soup

Cooking Time: 30 minutes | Serving: 4

Ingredients:

- ❖ 1 can low sodium diced tomatoes.
- ❖ Quinoa
- ❖ Vegetable broth
- ❖ Fresh basil leaves
- ❖ Carrots, diced.

Instructions:

1. Combine tomatoes, quinoa, and broth in a pot. Bring to a boil.
2. Add diced carrots and simmer until quinoa is cooked.
3. Stir in fresh basil before serving.

Nutritional Information:

160 calories, 25g carbs, 8g protein, 3g fat, 5g fiber.

Indulge in a flavorful tomato and quinoa soup, offering a burst of antioxidants and heart-healthy nutrients.

Chicken and Vegetable Barley Soup

Cooking Time: 50 minutes | Serving: 4

Ingredients:

- ❖ Chicken breast, diced.
- ❖ Barley
- ❖ Low-sodium chicken broth
- ❖ Mixed vegetables (carrots, peas, celery)
- ❖ Fresh thyme

Instructions:

1. Sauté diced chicken until cooked.
2. Add barley, vegetables, and broth. Simmer until barley is tender.
3. Garnish with fresh thyme before serving.

Nutritional Information:

220 calories, 30g carbs, 20g protein, 2g fat, 7g fiber.

Savor the wholesome goodness of chicken and barley, a comforting soup loaded with protein and heart-friendly grains.

Spinach and White Bean Soup

Cooking Time: 40 minutes | Serving: 4

Ingredients:

- ❖ White beans canned and drained.
- ❖ Fresh spinach
- ❖ Low-sodium vegetable broth
- ❖ Garlic, onion, carrots
- ❖ Italian seasoning

Instructions:

1. Sauté garlic, onion, and carrots until softened.
2. Add beans, broth, and Italian seasoning. Simmer until flavors meld.
3. Stir in fresh spinach before serving.

Nutritional Information:

190 calories, 30g carbs, 10g protein, 1g fat, 9g fiber.

Relish a nutrient-packed spinach and white bean soup, offering a blend of vitamins, minerals, and heart-healthy fiber.

Butternut Squash and Apple Soup

Cooking Time: 35 minutes | Serving: 4

Ingredients:

- ❖ Butternut squash peeled and diced.
- ❖ Apples peeled and chopped.
- ❖ Low-sodium vegetable broth
- ❖ Onion, nutmeg, cinnamon
- ❖ Greek yogurt (optional, for garnish)

Instructions:

1. Sauté onion, add squash, apples, broth, and spices. Simmer until tender.
2. Blend until smooth. Garnish with a dollop of Greek yogurt if desired.

Nutritional Information:

150 calories, 35g carbs, 3g protein, 1g fat, 7g fiber.

Embrace the sweetness of butternut squash and apples in this heartwarming soup, rich in antioxidants and vitamins.

Minestrone Soup with Whole Wheat Pasta

Cooking Time: 40 minutes | Serving: 4

Ingredients:

- ❖ Whole wheat pasta
- ❖ Cannellini beans canned and drained.
- ❖ Tomatoes, diced.
- ❖ Mixed vegetables (zucchini, carrots, green beans)
- ❖ Low-sodium vegetable broth
- ❖ Italian seasoning

Instructions:

1. Cook pasta separately. In a pot, combine vegetables, beans, broth, and seasoning.
2. Simmer until vegetables are tender.
3. Add cooked pasta before serving.

Nutritional Information:

220 calories, 40g carbs, 10g protein, 2g fat, 8g fiber.

Delight in the Italian flavors of this minestrone soup, featuring whole wheat pasta for added heart-healthy benefits.

Salmon and Kale Chowder

Cooking Time: 35 minutes | Serving: 4

Ingredients:

- ❖ Salmon fillet, flaked.
- ❖ Kale, chopped.
- ❖ Potatoes, diced.
- ❖ Low-sodium chicken broth
- ❖ Onion, garlic, dill
- ❖ Low-fat milk

Instructions:

1. Sauté onion and garlic. Add potatoes, broth, and dill. Simmer until potatoes are tender.
2. Add flaked salmon and kale. Cook until kale is wilted.
3. Stir in low-fat milk before serving.

Nutritional Information:

250 calories, 30g carbs, 20g protein, 5g fat, 6g fiber.

Indulge in the omega-3 goodness of salmon and the nutrient-packed kale in this heart-healthy chowder.

Beet and Carrot Ginger Soup

Cooking Time: 30 minutes | Serving: 4

Ingredients:

- ❖ Beets peeled and chopped.
- ❖ Carrots, chopped.
- ❖ Low-sodium vegetable broth
- ❖ Fresh ginger, grated.
- ❖ Coconut milk (optional)

Instructions:

1. Boil beets and carrots until tender. Blend with ginger and broth.
2. Return to heat, add coconut milk if desired, and simmer.
3. Garnish with a sprinkle of fresh ginger before serving.

Nutritional Information:

160 calories, 25g carbs, 3g protein, 5g fat, 7g fiber.

Savor the vibrant colors and antioxidants of beets and carrots in this unique and heart-healthy soup.

Turkey and Brown Rice Soup

Cooking Time: 45 minutes | Serving: 4

Ingredients:

- ❖ Ground turkey
- ❖ Brown rice, cooked.
- ❖ Low-sodium chicken broth
- ❖ Carrots, celery, onion
- ❖ Sage, thyme

Instructions:

1. Brown ground turkey. Add chopped vegetables, broth, and herbs. Simmer.
2. Stir in cooked brown rice before serving.

Nutritional Information:

230 calories, 25g carbs, 20g protein, 5g fat, 6g fiber.

Enjoy a hearty and protein-packed turkey and brown rice soup, perfect for supporting heart health and providing lasting energy.

Artichoke and Spinach Soup

Cooking Time: 25 minutes | Serving: 4

Ingredients:

- ❖ Artichoke hearts canned and drained.
- ❖ Fresh spinach
- ❖ Low-sodium vegetable broth
- ❖ Onion, garlic, nutmeg
- ❖ Greek yogurt (optional, for garnish)

Instructions:

1. Sauté onion and garlic. Add artichoke hearts, broth, and nutmeg. Simmer.
2. Add fresh spinach and cook until wilted.
3. Garnish with a dollop of Greek yogurt if desired.

Nutritional Information:

180 calories, 20g carbs, 6g protein, 3g fat, 7g fiber.

Indulge in the goodness of artichokes and spinach, creating a light and heart-healthy soup for a delightful meal.

These diverse and flavorful heart-healthy soup recipes are not just nourishing but also a testament to the joy of savoring wholesome ingredients. Designed to promote cardiovascular health, each soup brings a unique blend of nutrients and tastes. Warm your heart and body with these comforting bowls, reminding us that taking care of our hearts can be a delicious journey.

CHAPTER 5

SENSATIONAL SALADS

Grilled Chicken and Berry Salad

Prep Time: 20 minutes | Serving: 2

Ingredients:

- ❖ Grilled chicken breast
- ❖ Mixed berries (strawberries, blueberries)
- ❖ Mixed greens
- ❖ Feta cheese
- ❖ Balsamic vinaigrette

Instructions:

1. Slice grilled chicken and arrange on a bed of mixed greens.
2. Add fresh berries and crumbled feta cheese.
3. Drizzle with balsamic vinaigrette.

Nutritional Information:

250 calories, 15g carbs, 25g protein, 10g fat, 5g fiber.

Savor the sweetness of berries and the protein punch of grilled chicken in this refreshing and nutrient-packed salad.

Quinoa and Vegetable Salad

Prep Time: 25 minutes | Serving: 4

Ingredients:

- ❖ Cooked quinoa
- ❖ Cherry tomatoes, halved.
- ❖ Cucumber, diced.
- ❖ Avocado, cubed.
- ❖ Fresh basil
- ❖ Lemon vinaigrette

Instructions:

1. Mix quinoa with tomatoes, cucumber, and avocado.
2. Toss in fresh basil and drizzle with lemon vinaigrette.

Nutritional Information:

220 calories, 30g carbs, 7g protein, 10g fat, 5g fiber.

Elevate your salad game with the wholesome goodness of quinoa, paired with a medley of fresh vegetables.

Shrimp and Mango Salad

Prep Time: 15 minutes | Serving: 2

Ingredients:

- ❖ Grilled shrimp
- ❖ Romaine lettuce
- ❖ Mango, sliced.
- ❖ Red onion thinly sliced.
- ❖ Lime dressing

Instructions:

1. Arrange grilled shrimp on a bed of romaine lettuce.
2. Add sliced mango and red onion.
3. Drizzle with zesty lime dressing.

Nutritional Information:

180 calories, 20g carbs, 20g protein, 3g fat, 4g fiber.

Indulge in the tropical flavors of shrimp and mango, creating a light and satisfying salad for a delightful meal.

Chickpea and Greek Salad

Prep Time: 15 minutes | Serving: 3

Ingredients:

- ❖ Canned chickpeas, drained.
- ❖ Cherry tomatoes, halved.
- ❖ Cucumber, diced.
- ❖ Kalamata olives
- ❖ Feta cheese
- ❖ Greek dressing

Instructions:

Combine chickpeas, tomatoes, cucumber, olives, and feta.

Toss with Greek dressing until well coated.

Nutritional Information:

230 calories, 25g carbs, 10g protein, 10g fat, 6g fiber.

Enjoy the Mediterranean goodness of chickpeas, olives, and feta in this vibrant and flavorful Greek salad.

Asian Sesame Tofu Salad

Prep Time: 30 minutes | Serving: 2

Ingredients:

- ❖ Baked tofu, cubed.
- ❖ Napa cabbage, shredded.
- ❖ Carrots, julienned.
- ❖ Edamame
- ❖ Sesame ginger dressing

Instructions:

1. Combine tofu, cabbage, carrots, and edamame.
2. Toss with sesame ginger dressing for an Asian-inspired delight.

Nutritional Information:

210 calories, 15g carbs, 15g protein, 12g fat, 7g fiber.

Explore the fusion of flavors with this Asian sesame tofu salad, showcasing the versatility of tofu in a delicious way.

Spinach and Walnut Salad with Raspberry Vinaigrette

Prep Time: 15 minutes | Serving: 2

Ingredients:

- ❖ Fresh spinach leaves
- ❖ Walnuts, chopped.
- ❖ Feta cheese, crumbled.
- ❖ Fresh raspberries
- ❖ Raspberry vinaigrette

Instructions:

1. Toss spinach with walnuts, feta, and fresh raspberries.
2. Drizzle with a sweet and tangy raspberry vinaigrette.

Nutritional Information:

230 calories, 15g carbs, 8g protein, 18g fat, 6g fiber.

Indulge in the antioxidant-rich goodness of fresh berries and the crunch of walnuts in this delightful and nutritious salad.

Roasted Vegetable and Quinoa Salad

Prep Time: 30 minutes | Serving: 4

Ingredients:

- ❖ Roasted vegetables (bell peppers, zucchini, cherry tomatoes)
- ❖ Cooked quinoa
- ❖ Mixed greens
- ❖ Goat cheese
- ❖ Balsamic glaze

Instructions:

1. Combine roasted vegetables with quinoa on a bed of mixed greens.
2. Sprinkle with goat cheese and drizzle with balsamic glaze.

Nutritional Information:

240 calories, 30g carbs, 10g protein, 8g fat, 6g fiber.

Savor the medley of flavors and textures in this roasted vegetable and quinoa salad, creating a hearty and satisfying meal.

Tuna and Avocado Salad

Prep Time: 20 minutes | Serving: 2

Ingredients:

- ❖ Canned tuna, drained.
- ❖ Mixed greens
- ❖ Avocado, sliced.
- ❖ Cherry tomatoes, halved.
- ❖ Lemon herb dressing

Instructions:

1. Flake tuna over a bed of mixed greens.
2. Add sliced avocado and cherry tomatoes.
3. Drizzle with a refreshing lemon herb dressing.

Nutritional Information:

210 calories, 15g carbs, 20g protein, 10g fat, 5g fiber.

Enjoy the heart-healthy omega-3s in tuna and the creamy goodness of avocado in this protein-packed salad.

Mediterranean Quinoa Salad

Prep Time: 25 minutes | Serving: 4

Ingredients:

- ❖ Quinoa, cooked.
- ❖ Cucumber, diced.
- ❖ Cherry tomatoes, halved.
- ❖ Kalamata olives, sliced.
- ❖ Feta cheese
- ❖ Greek dressing

Instructions:

1. Mix cooked quinoa with cucumber, tomatoes, olives, and feta.
2. Toss with a generous amount of Greek dressing.

Nutritional Information:

220 calories, 30g carbs, 8g protein, 8g fat, 5g fiber.

Delight in the flavors of the Mediterranean with this quinoa salad, a fusion of wholesome grains and vibrant vegetables.

Caprese Salad with Balsamic Glaze

Prep Time: 15 minutes | Serving: 2

Ingredients:

- ❖ Fresh mozzarella, sliced.
- ❖ Tomatoes, sliced.
- ❖ Fresh basil leaves
- ❖ Balsamic glaze
- ❖ Olive oil (optional)

Instructions:

1. Alternate slices of mozzarella, tomatoes, and basil on a plate.
2. Drizzle with balsamic glaze (and olive oil if desired).

Nutritional Information:

180 calories, 10g carbs, 10g protein, 12g fat, 3g fiber.

Elevate simplicity with the classic Caprese salad, celebrating the harmony of fresh ingredients and balsamic sweetness.

These sensational salads offer a symphony of flavors and textures, showcasing the diversity and joy that healthy eating can bring. Each salad is a testament to the idea that nutritious meals can be both satisfying and delicious. Embrace the goodness of fresh produce, lean proteins, and vibrant dressings, making each bite a celebration of well-being and vitality.

CHAPTER 6

FLAVORFUL MAIN DISHES

Lemon Herb Baked Salmon

Cooking Time: 20 minutes | Serving: 2

Ingredients:

- ❖ Salmon fillets
- ❖ Lemon
- ❖ Fresh herbs (parsley, dill)
- ❖ Olive oil
- ❖ Garlic powder

Instructions:

1. Place salmon on a baking sheet, drizzle with olive oil, and sprinkle with herbs and garlic powder.
2. Bake until salmon is cooked through.
3. Squeeze fresh lemon juice before serving.

Nutritional Information:

250 calories, 2g carbs, 25g protein, 15g fat, 1g fiber.

Delight in the simplicity of this lemon herb salmon, a flavorful dish rich in omega-3s for heart and brain health.

Mushroom and Spinach Stuffed Chicken Breast

Cooking Time: 30 minutes | Serving: 2

Ingredients:

- ❖ Chicken breasts
- ❖ Mushrooms, chopped.
- ❖ Fresh spinach
- ❖ Garlic
- ❖ Low-sodium chicken broth

Instructions:

1. Sauté mushrooms, garlic, and spinach until wilted.
2. Cut a pocket into chicken breasts, stuff with the mushroom-spinach mixture.
3. Bake until chicken is cooked.

Nutritional Information:

220 calories, 5g carbs, 30g protein, 8g fat, 2g fiber.

Enjoy the culinary artistry of stuffed chicken, combining lean protein with nutrient-packed mushrooms and spinach.

Shrimp Stir-Fry with Vegetables

Cooking Time: 15 minutes | Serving: 2

Ingredients:

- ❖ Shrimp peeled and deveined.
- ❖ Mixed vegetables (bell peppers, broccoli, snap peas)
- ❖ Soy sauce (low sodium)
- ❖ Ginger, minced.
- ❖ Brown rice (optional, for serving)

Instructions:

1. Stir-fry shrimp and vegetables in a wok with soy sauce and minced ginger.
2. Serve over brown rice if desired.

Nutritional Information:

230 calories, 20g carbs, 25g protein, 5g fat, 4g fiber.

Dive into the flavors of this quick and easy shrimp stir-fry, packed with colorful veggies and lean protein.

Turkey and Vegetable Skewers

Cooking Time: 20 minutes | Serving: 2

Ingredients:

- ❖ Ground turkey
- ❖ Bell peppers, onions, cherry tomatoes (for skewers)
- ❖ Olive oil
- ❖ Italian seasoning

Instructions:

1. Mix ground turkey with Italian seasoning, shape into skewers with vegetables.
2. Grill until turkey is cooked and veggies are tender.
3. Drizzle with olive oil before serving.

Nutritional Information:

210 calories, 15g carbs, 25g protein, 8g fat, 3g fiber.

Savor the simplicity of turkey skewers, a lean and flavorful option for a satisfying main dish.

Eggplant Parmesan

Cooking Time: 40 minutes | Serving: 2

Ingredients:

- ❖ Eggplant, sliced.
- ❖ Whole wheat breadcrumbs
- ❖ Marinara sauce (low sodium)
- ❖ Mozzarella cheese, shredded.
- ❖ Fresh basil

Instructions:

1. Coat eggplant slices in whole wheat breadcrumbs.
2. Bake until crispy, then layer with marinara sauce and mozzarella.
3. Bake until cheese is melted, garnish with fresh basil.

Nutritional Information:

230 calories, 25g carbs, 15g protein, 10g fat, 7g fiber.

Relish the Italian flavors of this healthier Eggplant Parmesan, showcasing the versatility of this nutrient-rich vegetable.

Lemon Garlic Herb Grilled Chicken

Cooking Time: 25 minutes | Serving: 2

Ingredients:

- ❖ Chicken thighs
- ❖ Lemon
- ❖ Garlic, minced.
- ❖ Fresh herbs (rosemary, thyme)
- ❖ Olive oil

Instructions:

1. Marinate chicken in a mixture of lemon juice, minced garlic, and fresh herbs.
2. Grill until chicken is cooked through.
3. Drizzle with olive oil before serving.

Nutritional Information:

260 calories, 1g carbs, 30g protein, 15g fat, 0g fiber.

Elevate your grilled chicken with the zesty freshness of lemon and a medley of aromatic herbs.

Sweet Potato and Black Bean Chili

Cooking Time: 30 minutes | Serving: 4

Ingredients:

- ❖ Sweet potatoes, diced.
- ❖ Black beans canned and drained.
- ❖ Onion, diced.
- ❖ Chili powder, cumin
- ❖ Low-sodium vegetable broth

Instructions:

1. Sauté onions until soft, add sweet potatoes, beans, and spices.
2. Pour in vegetable broth and simmer until sweet potatoes are tender.

Nutritional Information:

240 calories, 40g carbs, 10g protein, 3g fat, 8g fiber.

Warm your soul with this hearty sweet potato and black bean chili, a fiber-rich and satisfying dish.

Lemon Dill Baked Cod

Cooking Time: 20 minutes | Serving: 2

Ingredients:

- ❖ Cod fillets
- ❖ Lemon
- ❖ Fresh dill
- ❖ Garlic powder
- ❖ Olive oil

Instructions:

1. Place cod on a baking sheet, season with garlic powder, dill, and lemon slices.
2. Bake until cod is flaky.
3. Drizzle with olive oil before serving.

Nutritional Information:

190 calories, 1g carbs, 25g protein, 8g fat, 0g fiber.

Enjoy the lightness of baked cod infused with the citrusy brightness of lemon and the aromatic touch of dill.

Mediterranean Chickpea Salad Bowl

Prep Time: 15 minutes | Serving: 2

Ingredients:

- ❖ Canned chickpeas, drained.
- ❖ Cucumber, diced.
- ❖ Cherry tomatoes, halved.
- ❖ Feta cheese, crumbled.
- ❖ Kalamata olives, sliced.
- ❖ Olive oil, balsamic vinegar

Instructions:

1. Mix chickpeas, cucumber, tomatoes, feta, and olives.
2. Drizzle with olive oil and balsamic vinegar.

Nutritional Information:

250 calories, 30g carbs, 12g protein, 10g fat, 8g fiber.

Relish the flavors of the Mediterranean in this vibrant chickpea salad bowl, a refreshing and nutrient-packed delight.

Teriyaki Tofu Stir-Fry

Cooking Time: 25 minutes | Serving: 3

Ingredients:

- ❖ Extra-firm tofu, cubed.
- ❖ Mixed vegetables (broccoli, bell peppers, carrots)
- ❖ Low-sodium teriyaki sauce
- ❖ Brown rice (optional, for serving)

Instructions:

1. Sauté tofu until golden, add mixed vegetables and teriyaki sauce.
2. Stir-fry until veggies are tender.
3. Serve over brown rice if desired.

Nutritional Information:

230 calories, 25g carbs, 15g protein, 10g fat, 5g fiber.

Embrace the savory goodness of teriyaki tofu stir-fry, a plant-based option that's both flavorful and satisfying.

Baked Zucchini Boats with Turkey

Cooking Time: 30 minutes | Serving: 2

Ingredients:

- ❖ Zucchini, halved.
- ❖ Ground turkey
- ❖ Tomato sauce (low sodium)
- ❖ Italian seasoning
- ❖ Parmesan cheese, grated.

Instructions:

1. Hollow out zucchini halves.
2. Brown ground turkey, mix with tomato sauce and Italian seasoning.
3. Fill zucchini with the turkey mixture, sprinkle with Parmesan.
4. Bake until zucchini is tender.

Nutritional Information:

220 calories, 15g carbs, 20g protein, 10g fat, 4g fiber.

Savor the Italian-inspired flavors of these zucchini boats, a low-carb option filled with protein.

Broccoli and Cheddar Stuffed Chicken Breast

Cooking Time: 35 minutes | Serving: 2

Ingredients:

- ❖ Chicken breasts
- ❖ Broccoli florets, steamed.
- ❖ Cheddar cheese, shredded.
- ❖ Dijon mustard
- ❖ Garlic powder

Instructions:

1. Cut a pocket into chicken breasts.
2. Stuff with steamed broccoli and cheddar.
3. Season with garlic powder and bake until chicken is cooked.

Nutritional Information:

260 calories, 5g carbs, 30g protein, 12g fat, 2g fiber.

Indulge in the comforting combination of broccoli and cheddar in this stuffed chicken breast.

Spaghetti Squash Primavera

Cooking Time: 40 minutes | Serving: 3

Ingredients:

- ❖ Spaghetti squash, roasted.
- ❖ Mixed vegetables (zucchini, cherry tomatoes, bell peppers)
- ❖ Olive oil
- ❖ Garlic, minced.
- ❖ Fresh basil

Instructions:

1. Roast spaghetti squash, scrape into "noodles."
2. Sauté mixed vegetables and garlic in olive oil.
3. Toss with spaghetti squash, garnish with fresh basil.

Nutritional Information:

180 calories, 20g carbs, 3g protein, 10g fat, 5g fiber.

Enjoy a lighter take on pasta with this spaghetti squash primavera, bursting with colorful vegetables.

Herb-Crusted Tilapia

Cooking Time: 20 minutes | Serving: 2

Ingredients:

- ❖ Tilapia fillets
- ❖ Whole wheat breadcrumbs
- ❖ Fresh herbs (parsley, thyme)
- ❖ Lemon
- ❖ Olive oil

Instructions:

1. Coat tilapia with a mixture of breadcrumbs and chopped herbs.
2. Drizzle with olive oil and bake until fish is flaky.
3. Squeeze fresh lemon juice before serving.

Nutritional Information:

190 calories, 10g carbs, 25g protein, 7g fat, 2g fiber.

Elevate the mild flavor of tilapia with a zesty herb crust, creating a light and delightful main dish.

Cauliflower Fried Rice with Shrimp

Cooking Time: 25 minutes | Serving: 3

Ingredients:

- ❖ Cauliflower rice
- ❖ Shrimp peeled and deveined.
- ❖ Mixed vegetables (peas, carrots, corn)
- ❖ Soy sauce (low sodium)
- ❖ Scrambled eggs

Instructions:

1. Sauté shrimp and vegetables in a pan with soy sauce.
2. Add cauliflower rice and scrambled eggs, stir-fry until heated through.

Nutritional Information:

220 calories, 15g carbs, 20g protein, 10g fat, 5g fiber.

Enjoy the comfort of fried rice without the carbs with this cauliflower fried rice featuring succulent shrimp.

Lentil and Vegetable Curry

Cooking Time: 40 minutes | Serving: 4

Ingredients:

- ❖ Lentils, cooked.
- ❖ Mixed vegetables (peppers, peas, carrots)
- ❖ Coconut milk (light)
- ❖ Curry powder, cumin
- ❖ Garlic, minced.

Instructions:

1. Sauté garlic, add mixed vegetables, lentils, coconut milk, and spices.
2. Simmer until vegetables are tender.

Nutritional Information:

240 calories, 30g carbs, 12g protein, 8g fat, 8g fiber.

Delight in the aromatic and flavorful experience of lentil and vegetable curry, a comforting and nutritious choice.

Baked Chicken with Lemon and Rosemary

Cooking Time: 35 minutes | Serving: 2

Ingredients:

- ❖ Chicken thighs
- ❖ Lemon
- ❖ Fresh rosemary
- ❖ Garlic powder
- ❖ Olive oil

Instructions:

1. Marinate chicken with olive oil, lemon juice, rosemary, and garlic powder.
2. Bake until chicken is golden and cooked through.

Nutritional Information:

250 calories, 1g carbs, 30g protein, 15g fat, 0g fiber.

Enjoy a burst of citrus and herb flavors with this baked chicken, a simple yet satisfying dish.

Veggie-Packed Turkey Meatballs

Cooking Time: 30 minutes | Serving: 4

Ingredients:

- ❖ Ground turkey
- ❖ Grated zucchini
- ❖ Whole wheat breadcrumbs
- ❖ Tomato sauce (low sodium)
- ❖ Italian seasoning

Instructions:

1. Mix ground turkey with grated zucchini, breadcrumbs, and Italian seasoning.
2. Form into meatballs and bake until cooked through.
3. Serve over whole wheat pasta with tomato sauce.

Nutritional Information:

220 calories, 20g carbs, 25g protein, 8g fat, 4g fiber.

Transform traditional meatballs into a nutritious delight with the addition of zucchini for a veggie boost.

Stuffed Bell Peppers with Quinoa and Black Beans

Cooking Time: 45 minutes | Serving: 4

Ingredients:

- ❖ Bell peppers, halved.
- ❖ Quinoa, cooked.
- ❖ Black beans canned and drained.
- ❖ Corn kernels
- ❖ Salsa (low sodium)

Instructions:

1. Mix cooked quinoa, black beans, corn, and salsa.
2. Stuff bell peppers with the quinoa mixture.
3. Bake until peppers are tender.

Nutritional Information:

260 calories, 40g carbs, 10g protein, 5g fat, 8g fiber.

Experience a burst of flavors with these stuffed bell peppers, combining the goodness of quinoa and black beans.

Balsamic Glazed Chicken with Roasted Vegetables

Cooking Time: 40 minutes | Serving: 2

Ingredients:

- ❖ Chicken breasts
- ❖ Mixed vegetables (brussels sprouts, carrots, red onion)
- ❖ Balsamic glaze
- ❖ Olive oil
- ❖ Thyme, dried

Instructions:

1. Coat chicken with balsamic glaze, thyme, and olive oil.
2. Roast chicken and mixed vegetables until cooked through.

Nutritional Information:

240 calories, 25g carbs, 30g protein, 8g fat, 6g fiber.

Relish the savory-sweet combination of balsamic-glazed chicken paired with perfectly roasted vegetables.

CHAPTER 7

DELICIOUS DESSERTS

Fresh Berry Parfait

Prep Time: 15 minutes | Serving: 2

Ingredients:

- ❖ Mixed berries (strawberries, blueberries, raspberries)
- ❖ Greek yogurt (unsweetened)
- ❖ Honey (optional)
- ❖ Granola (low sodium)

Instructions:

1. Layer berries and Greek yogurt in a glass.
2. Drizzle with honey if desired and top with granola.

Nutritional Information:

180 calories, 30g carbs, 10g protein, 3g fat, 5g fiber.

Indulge in the natural sweetness of fresh berries and the creaminess of Greek yogurt for a guilt-free and delightful dessert.

Baked Apples with Cinnamon and Walnuts

Cooking Time: 30 minutes | Serving: 2

Ingredients:

- ❖ Apples cored and halved.
- ❖ Cinnamon
- ❖ Walnuts, chopped.
- ❖ Maple syrup (optional)

Instructions:

1. Place apple halves on a baking sheet.
2. Sprinkle with cinnamon and walnuts.
3. Drizzle with maple syrup if desired and bake until apples are tender.

Nutritional Information:

160 calories, 25g carbs, 3g protein, 7g fat, 5g fiber.

Enjoy the warmth and aroma of baked apples, a comforting and nutritious dessert option with a hint of cinnamon.

Chia Seed Pudding with Mango

Prep Time: 5 minutes | Chilling Time: 4 hours | Serving: 2

Ingredients:

- ❖ Chia seeds
- ❖ Almond milk (unsweetened)
- ❖ Vanilla extract
- ❖ Mango, diced.

Instructions:

1. Mix chia seeds, almond milk, and vanilla extract in a bowl.
2. Refrigerate for at least 4 hours or overnight.
3. Top with diced mango before serving.

Nutritional Information:

200 calories, 15g carbs, 5g protein, 10g fat, 8g fiber.

Savor the simplicity of chia seed pudding, a versatile and fiber-rich dessert that pairs perfectly with sweet mango.

Banana-Oat Cookies

Prep Time: 15 minutes | Baking Time: 12 minutes | Serving: 2

Ingredients:

- ❖ Ripe bananas, mashed.
- ❖ Rolled oats.
- ❖ Cinnamon
- ❖ Nuts (walnuts or almonds), chopped.

Instructions:

1. Mix mashed bananas, oats, cinnamon, and chopped nuts.
2. Scoop onto a baking sheet and bake until golden.

Nutritional Information:

160 calories, 30g carbs, 5g protein, 4g fat, 4g fiber.

Embrace the natural sweetness of ripe bananas in these wholesome and easy-to-make oat cookies.

Greek Yogurt with Honey and Almonds

Prep Time: 5 minutes | Serving: 2

Ingredients:

- ❖ Greek yogurt (unsweetened)
- ❖ Honey
- ❖ Almonds, sliced.

Instructions:

1. Spoon Greek yogurt into serving bowls.
2. Drizzle with honey and sprinkle with sliced almonds.

Nutritional Information:

180 calories, 15g carbs, 15g protein, 8g fat, 2g fiber.

Transform plain Greek yogurt into a luscious dessert with the natural sweetness of honey and the crunch of almonds.

Poached Pears with Vanilla Yogurt

Cooking Time: 20 minutes | Serving: 2

Ingredients:

- ❖ Pears peeled and halved.
- ❖ Water
- ❖ Vanilla extract
- ❖ Greek yogurt (unsweetened)

Instructions:

1. Poach pears in water with vanilla extract until tender.
2. Serve with a dollop of Greek yogurt.

Nutritional Information:

200 calories, 40g carbs, 10g protein, 2g fat, 8g fiber.

Elevate the elegance of poached pears with a touch of vanilla, creating a simple and refined dessert.

Dark Chocolate-Dipped Strawberries

Prep Time: 15 minutes | Serving: 2

Ingredients:

- ❖ Strawberries washed and dried.
- ❖ Dark chocolate (low sodium)
- ❖ Almonds finely chopped.

Instructions:

1. Melt dark chocolate in a bowl.
2. Dip strawberries into melted chocolate and sprinkle with chopped almonds.
3. Allow to cool until chocolate hardens.

Nutritional Information:

160 calories, 20g carbs, 2g protein, 10g fat, 5g fiber.

Indulge in the classic combination of dark chocolate and strawberries, creating a decadent yet heart-healthy treat.

Pineapple Coconut Sorbet

Prep Time: 10 minutes | Freezing Time: 4 hours | Serving: 2

Ingredients:

- ❖ Pineapple, frozen
- ❖ Coconut milk (unsweetened)
- ❖ Lime juice

Instructions:

1. Blend frozen pineapple, coconut milk, and lime juice until smooth.
2. Freeze for at least 4 hours before serving.

Nutritional Information:

140 calories, 25g carbs, 1g protein, 6g fat, 3g fiber.

Cool down with this tropical delight—pineapple coconut sorbet, a refreshing and dairy-free dessert.

Almond Flour Blueberry Muffins

Prep Time: 15 minutes | Baking Time: 20 minutes | Serving: 2

Ingredients:

- ❖ Almond flour
- ❖ Eggs
- ❖ Baking powder
- ❖ Blueberries
- ❖ Vanilla extract

Instructions:

1. Mix almond flour, eggs, baking powder, and vanilla extract.
2. Gently fold in blueberries.
3. Bake in muffin cups until golden.

Nutritional Information:

180 calories, 10g carbs, 7g protein, 12g fat, 3g fiber.

Enjoy the goodness of almond flour in these blueberry muffins, a gluten-free and wholesome dessert option.

Cinnamon-Spiced Baked Pears

Prep Time: 10 minutes | Baking Time: 25 minutes | Serving: 2

Ingredients:

- ❖ Pears halved and cored.
- ❖ Cinnamon
- ❖ Walnuts, chopped.
- ❖ Maple syrup (optional)

Instructions:

1. Place pear halves on a baking sheet.
2. Sprinkle with cinnamon and chopped walnuts.
3. Drizzle with maple syrup if desired and bake until pears are soft.

Nutritional Information:

190 calories, 30g carbs, 3g protein, 8g fat, 6g fiber.

Embrace the warmth of cinnamon and the nutty crunch of walnuts in these comforting baked pears.

CHAPTER 8
21 DAY MEAL PLAN

Day 1:

- ❖ Breakfast: Avocado Banana Smoothie
- ❖ Lunch: Mediterranean Chickpea Salad Bowl
- ❖ Dinner: Lemon Herb Baked Salmon
- ❖ Dessert: Fresh Berry Parfait

Day 2:

- ❖ Breakfast: Chia Seed Pudding with Mango
- ❖ Lunch: Shrimp Stir-Fry with Vegetables
- ❖ Dinner: Mushroom and Spinach Stuffed Chicken Breast
- ❖ Dessert: Baked Apples with Cinnamon and Walnuts

Day 3:

- ❖ Breakfast: Greek Yogurt with Honey and Almonds
- ❖ Lunch: Sweet Potato and Black Bean Chili
- ❖ Dinner: Teriyaki Tofu Stir-Fry
- ❖ Dessert: Dark Chocolate-Dipped Strawberries

Day 4:

- ❖ Breakfast: Banana-Oat Cookies
- ❖ Lunch: Lentil and Vegetable Curry
- ❖ Dinner: Balsamic Glazed Chicken with Roasted Vegetables
- ❖ Dessert: Blueberry Almond Smoothie Bowl

Day 5:

- ❖ Breakfast: Baked Zucchini Boats with Turkey
- ❖ Lunch: Spaghetti Squash Primavera
- ❖ Dinner: Herb-Crusted Tilapia
- ❖ Dessert: Greek Yogurt with Honey and Almonds

Day 6:

- ❖ Breakfast: Lemon Garlic Herb Grilled Chicken
- ❖ Lunch: Turkey and Vegetable Skewers
- ❖ Dinner: Eggplant Parmesan
- ❖ Dessert: Raspberry Almond Protein Smoothie

Day 7:

- ❖ Breakfast: Broccoli and Cheddar Stuffed Chicken Breast
- ❖ Lunch: Lemon Dill Baked Cod
- ❖ Dinner: Creamy Avocado Banana Smoothie
- ❖ Dessert: Peach and Banana Sunrise Smoothie

Day 8:

- ❖ Breakfast: Lemon Herb Baked Salmon
- ❖ Lunch: Baked Chicken with Lemon and Rosemary
- ❖ Dinner: Veggie-Packed Turkey Meatballs
- ❖ Dessert: Cherry Almond Antioxidant Smoothie

Day 9:

- ❖ Breakfast: Teriyaki Tofu Stir-Fry
- ❖ Lunch: Mediterranean Chickpea Salad Bowl
- ❖ Dinner: Stuffed Bell Peppers with Quinoa and Black Beans
- ❖ Dessert: Cinnamon-Spiced Baked Pears

Day 10:

- ❖ Breakfast: Mushroom and Spinach Stuffed Chicken Breast
- ❖ Lunch: Lemon Dill Baked Cod
- ❖ Dinner: Balsamic Glazed Chicken with Roasted Vegetables
- ❖ Dessert: Greek Yogurt with Honey and Almonds

Day 11:

- ❖ Breakfast: Eggplant Parmesan
- ❖ Lunch: Lentil and Vegetable Curry
- ❖ Dinner: Sweet Potato and Black Bean Chili
- ❖ Dessert: Fresh Berry Parfait

Day 12:

- ❖ Breakfast: Banana-Oat Cookies
- ❖ Lunch: Shrimp Stir-Fry with Vegetables
- ❖ Dinner: Herb-Crusted Tilapia
- ❖ Dessert: Blueberry Almond Smoothie Bowl

Day 13:

- ❖ Breakfast: Baked Zucchini Boats with Turkey
- ❖ Lunch: Spaghetti Squash Primavera
- ❖ Dinner: Lemon Garlic Herb Grilled Chicken
- ❖ Dessert: Raspberry Almond Protein Smoothie

Day 14:

- ❖ Breakfast: Broccoli and Cheddar Stuffed Chicken Breast
- ❖ Lunch: Dark Chocolate-Dipped Strawberries
- ❖ Dinner: Creamy Avocado Banana Smoothie
- ❖ Dessert: Peach and Banana Sunrise Smoothie

Day 15:

- ❖ Breakfast: Lemon Herb Baked Salmon
- ❖ Lunch: Baked Chicken with Lemon and Rosemary
- ❖ Dinner: Veggie-Packed Turkey Meatballs
- ❖ Dessert: Cherry Almond Antioxidant Smoothie

Day 16:

- ❖ Breakfast: Teriyaki Tofu Stir-Fry
- ❖ Lunch: Mediterranean Chickpea Salad Bowl
- ❖ Dinner: Stuffed Bell Peppers with Quinoa and Black Beans
- ❖ Dessert: Cinnamon-Spiced Baked Pears

Day 17:

- ❖ Breakfast: Mushroom and Spinach Stuffed Chicken Breast
- ❖ Lunch: Lemon Dill Baked Cod
- ❖ Dinner: Sweet Potato and Black Bean Chili
- ❖ Dessert: Greek Yogurt with Honey and Almonds

Day 18:

- ❖ Breakfast: Eggplant Parmesan
- ❖ Lunch: Lentil and Vegetable Curry
- ❖ Dinner: Lemon Garlic Herb Grilled Chicken
- ❖ Dessert: Fresh Berry Parfait

Day 19:

- ❖ Breakfast: Banana-Oat Cookies
- ❖ Lunch: Shrimp Stir-Fry with Vegetables
- ❖ Dinner: Herb-Crusted Tilapia
- ❖ Dessert: Blueberry Almond Smoothie Bowl

Day 20:

- ❖ Breakfast: Baked Zucchini Boats with Turkey
- ❖ Lunch: Spaghetti Squash Primavera
- ❖ Dinner: Lemon Dill Baked Cod
- ❖ Dessert: Raspberry Almond Protein Smoothie

Day 21:

- ❖ Breakfast: Broccoli and Cheddar Stuffed Chicken Breast
- ❖ Lunch: Dark Chocolate-Dipped Strawberries
- ❖ Dinner: Creamy Avocado Banana Smoothie
- ❖ Dessert: Peach and Banana Sunrise Smoothie

CONCLUSION

As we conclude our journey through the flavorful pages of "Low-Sodium Cookbook for Seniors," I want to express my heartfelt gratitude for joining me on this culinary adventure. Together, we've explored the art of crafting delicious, health-conscious meals that transcend the boundaries of traditional cookbooks.

In the tapestry of our stories, each recipe has played a unique role in transforming not just our meals but our entire approach to healthy living. From the zesty kick of the Citrus Berry Burst Smoothie to the comforting embrace of the Stuffed Bell Peppers with Quinoa and Black Beans, these recipes have become more than just instructions—they are gateways to a life rich in vitality and flavor.

As you venture into the world of " Low-Sodium Cookbook for Seniors," my hope is that you find inspiration in every dish, joy in every bite, and a renewed sense of well-being with each chapter turned. The journey toward a low-sodium lifestyle is not just a path to better health; it's an odyssey of self-discovery and a celebration of the beautiful connection between food and life.

I invite you to share your experiences, your triumphs, and even your challenges as you navigate this culinary landscape. Your feedback is not only welcomed but cherished. Did you discover a favorite recipe that became a staple in your kitchen? How did "Savoring Harmony" influence your health and daily routines? Your insights will not only enrich our community but will also guide the evolution of future editions.

Remember, our journey doesn't end here—it's a continuous exploration of the harmonious intersection of taste and well-being. Your feedback will shape the future of " Low-Sodium Cookbook for Seniors," ensuring that it remains a trusted companion on your culinary quest.

As you embark on this flavorful chapter of your life, savoring the harmonious notes of each recipe, I encourage you to share your thoughts, questions, and experiences. Let our community become a space where we exchange not just recipes but stories, where the love for wholesome, low-sodium meals becomes a shared passion.

Thank you for being a part of the "Savoring Harmony" family. May your kitchens be filled with the aroma of delicious possibilities, and may every meal be a celebration of health, joy, and the simple pleasures that make life truly extraordinary.

Here's to savoring the harmony of life—one delightful recipe at a time.

BONUS CHAPTER

10 HEALTY SMOOTHIES

Berry Bliss Smoothie

Prep Time: 5 minutes | Serving: 1

Ingredients:

- ❖ Mixed berries (strawberries, blueberries, raspberries)
- ❖ Greek yogurt (unsweetened)
- ❖ Spinach leaves
- ❖ Almond milk (unsweetened)
- ❖ Chia seeds

Instructions:

1. Blend berries, Greek yogurt, spinach, and almond milk until smooth.
2. Stir in chia seeds and blend for a few more seconds.

Nutritional Information:

180 calories, 20g carbs, 10g protein, 7g fat, 6g fiber.

Start your day with a burst of antioxidants and energy from this delightful and nutrient-packed berry smoothie.

Tropical Green Smoothie

Prep Time: 5 minutes | Serving: 1

Ingredients:

- ❖ Pineapple chunks
- ❖ Mango peeled and diced.
- ❖ Spinach leaves
- ❖ Coconut water
- ❖ Flaxseeds

Instructions:

1. Blend pineapple, mango, spinach, and coconut water until smooth.
2. Add flaxseeds and blend for an extra boost.

Nutritional Information:

200 calories, 30g carbs, 5g protein, 8g fat, 5g fiber.

Transport yourself to the tropics with this refreshing and hydrating tropical green smoothie.

Creamy Avocado Banana Smoothie

Prep Time: 5 minutes | Serving: 1

Ingredients:

- ❖ Avocado peeled and pitted.
- ❖ Banana
- ❖ Greek yogurt (unsweetened)
- ❖ Almond milk (unsweetened)
- ❖ Honey (optional)

Instructions:

1. Blend avocado, banana, Greek yogurt, and almond milk until creamy.
2. Add honey if desired and blend for a sweeter taste.

Nutritional Information:

220 calories, 25g carbs, 7g protein, 12g fat, 6g fiber.

Embrace the creaminess of avocado in this smoothie for a dose of healthy fats and a satisfying texture.

Citrus Berry Burst Smoothie

Prep Time: 5 minutes | Serving: 1

Ingredients:

- ❖ Orange, peeled.
- ❖ Mixed berries (strawberries, blueberries, raspberries)
- ❖ Greek yogurt (unsweetened)
- ❖ Water or coconut water
- ❖ Ice cubes

Instructions:

1. Blend orange, mixed berries, Greek yogurt, and water (or coconut water) until smooth.
2. Add ice cubes and blend for a refreshing kick.

Nutritional Information:

160 calories, 30g carbs, 8g protein, 2g fat, 5g fiber.

Revel in the zesty goodness of citrus paired with the vibrant flavors of mixed berries in this invigorating smoothie.

Kale and Pineapple Power Smoothie

Prep Time: 5 minutes | Serving: 1

Ingredients:

- ❖ Kale leaves, stems removed.
- ❖ Pineapple chunks
- ❖ Banana
- ❖ Coconut water
- ❖ Hemp seeds

Instructions:

1. Blend kale, pineapple, banana, and coconut water until smooth.
2. Add hemp seeds for an extra nutritional boost.

Nutritional Information:

190 calories, 30g carbs, 7g protein, 6g fat, 7g fiber.

Harness the power of kale and pineapple for a nutrient-dense smoothie that fuels your day.

Blueberry Almond Smoothie Bowl

Prep Time: 10 minutes | Serving: 1

Ingredients:

- ❖ Frozen blueberries
- ❖ Almond butter
- ❖ Almond milk (unsweetened)
- ❖ Rolled oats.
- ❖ Toppings: sliced almonds, chia seeds

Instructions:

1. Blend blueberries, almond butter, almond milk, and rolled oats until smooth.
2. Pour into a bowl and top with sliced almonds and chia seeds.

Nutritional Information:

240 calories, 30g carbs, 8g protein, 12g fat, 6g fiber.

Elevate your smoothie experience with a delicious and satisfying blueberry almond smoothie bowl.

Spinach and Mango Delight Smoothie

Prep Time: 5 minutes | Serving: 1

Ingredients:

- ❖ Fresh spinach leaves
- ❖ Mango peeled and diced.
- ❖ Greek yogurt (unsweetened)
- ❖ Coconut water
- ❖ Mint leaves (optional)

Instructions:

1. Blend spinach, mango, Greek yogurt, and coconut water until smooth.
2. Garnish with mint leaves for a refreshing twist.

Nutritional Information:

170 calories, 25g carbs, 8g protein, 5g fat, 4g fiber.

Combine the goodness of spinach and the tropical sweetness of mango in this vibrant and healthful smoothie.

Raspberry Almond Protein Smoothie

Prep Time: 5 minutes | Serving: 1

Ingredients:

- ❖ Raspberries
- ❖ Almond milk (unsweetened)
- ❖ Protein powder (unsweetened)
- ❖ Almonds, sliced.
- ❖ Ice cubes

Instructions:

1. Blend raspberries, almond milk, protein powder, and ice cubes until smooth.
2. Top with sliced almonds for added crunch.

Nutritional Information:

220 calories, 15g carbs, 20g protein, 10g fat, 6g fiber.

Boost your protein intake with this raspberry almond protein smoothie, perfect for post-workout recovery.

Peach and Banana Sunrise Smoothie

Prep Time: 5 minutes | Serving: 1

Ingredients:

- ❖ Peaches, sliced.
- ❖ Banana
- ❖ Orange juice (unsweetened)
- ❖ Yogurt (unsweetened)
- ❖ Flaxseeds

Instructions:

1. Blend peaches, banana, orange juice, and yogurt until smooth.
2. Add flaxseeds for a nutritional punch.

Nutritional Information:

190 calories, 35g carbs, 6g protein, 3g fat, 5g fiber.

Awaken your senses with the sweet combination of peaches and banana in this vibrant sunrise smoothie.

Cherry Almond Antioxidant Smoothie

Prep Time: 5 minutes | Serving: 1

Ingredients:

- ❖ Cherries, pitted.
- ❖ Almond milk (unsweetened)
- ❖ Greek yogurt (unsweetened)
- ❖ Honey (optional)
- ❖ Ice cubes

Instructions:

1. Blend cherries, almond milk, Greek yogurt, and ice cubes until smooth.
2. Add honey if additional sweetness is desired.

Nutritional Information:

210 calories, 30g carbs, 10g protein, 7g fat, 4g fiber.

Enjoy the antioxidant-rich goodness of cherries and the nutty notes of almonds in this delectable smoothie.

MEAL PLANNER JOURNAL

WEEKLY PLANNER

MONDAY	TUESDAY

WEDNESDAY	THURSDAY

FRIDAY	SATUREDAY

SUNDAY	NOTE

WEEKLY PLANNER

MONDAY

TUESDAY

WEDNESDAY

THURSDAY

FRIDAY

SATUREDAY

SUNDAY

NOTE

WEEKLY PLANNER

MONDAY	TUESDAY

WEDNESDAY	THURSDAY

FRIDAY	SATUREDAY

SUNDAY	NOTE

WEEKLY PLANNER

MONDAY

TUESDAY

WEDNESDAY

THURSDAY

FRIDAY

SATUREDAY

SUNDAY

NOTE

WEEKLY PLANNER

MONDAY	TUESDAY

WEDNESDAY	THURSDAY

FRIDAY	SATUREDAY

SUNDAY	NOTE

WEEKLY PLANNER

MONDAY	TUESDAY

WEDNESDAY	THURSDAY

FRIDAY	SATUREDAY

SUNDAY	NOTE

WEEKLY PLANNER

MONDAY	TUESDAY

WEDNESDAY	THURSDAY

FRIDAY	SATUREDAY

SUNDAY	NOTE

WEEKLY PLANNER

MONDAY	TUESDAY

WEDNESDAY	THURSDAY

FRIDAY	SATUREDAY

SUNDAY	NOTE

WEEKLY PLANNER

MONDAY	TUESDAY

WEDNESDAY	THURSDAY

FRIDAY	SATUREDAY

SUNDAY	NOTE

WEEKLY PLANNER

MONDAY	TUESDAY

WEDNESDAY	THURSDAY

FRIDAY	SATUREDAY

SUNDAY	NOTE